DIVERTICULOSIS MANAGEMENT DIET COOKBOOK

Delicious Recipes And Expert-Guidance For Digestive Health: Practical Strategies For Wellness Through Diet

DR. SHAYLA LEWIS

Table of Contents

DISCLAIMER

Write a brief complete Disclaimer for my diet cook book telling them that the author is not in any association with any company, business or individual and also this book is written by the authors knowledge and understanding

The information provided in this diet cookbook is based on the author's personal knowledge and understanding. The author is not affiliated with, endorsed by, or associated with any company, business, or individual. The recipes and dietary advice contained within this book are intended for informational purposes only. Readers should consult with a healthcare professional or a registered dietitian before making any significant changes to their diet or lifestyle. The author assumes no responsibility for any adverse effects that may result from the use or misuse of the information contained in this book.

CHAPTER ONE

Knowing What Diverticulosis Is

A prevalent disorder that affects the colon, more especially the large intestine, is diverticulosis. It happens when the intestinal lining develops tiny, protruding pouches called diverticula. Diverticulitis is a disorder that arises when diverticula become inflamed or infected, even though they may not cause symptoms on their own.

Diverticulosis: What is it?

These diverticula in the colon are a sign of diverticulosis. These pouches commonly appear where blood vessels pierce the muscular layer, which is a weak point in the colon wall. Diverticula come in different sizes and quantities, and they are frequently asymptomatic.

Diverticulosis is thought to be caused by a mix of variables, including age, diet, and genetics, though the precise cause is yet unknown. One of the main risk factors is regarded to be a diet poor in fiber. A low-fiber diet makes the stool tougher, which increases colonic pressure during bowel movements and can cause diverticula to form.

Obesity, inactivity, smoking, and some medications are additional risk factors. Diverticulosis is more common in elderly persons, therefore age also plays a part.

Typical symptoms

Typically, diverticulosis does not manifest any symptoms. However, some people could have symptoms including diarrhea, constipation, cramps, or bloating. These are frequently transient, mild symptoms.

In order to effectively manage diverticulosis, diet is essential. Constipation can be avoided and colon pressure can be decreased with a high-fiber diet, which also lowers the risk of diverticula formation and diverticulitis flare-ups. Fibre gives the stool more volume, which facilitates passage through the intestines.

Furthermore, avoiding or consuming specific foods in moderation might help prevent the exacerbation of symptoms and diverticulitis bouts. Foods heavy in red meat, saturated fats, and processed carbohydrates may be among them.

How this book can be useful

The Diverticulosis Management Diet Cookbook is intended to offer readers helpful advice and delectable meals that complement a diet suitable for diverticulosis sufferers. It attempts to provide people with diverticulosis the ability to make knowledgeable food decisions that can reduce symptoms, avoid problems, and enhance general health. This cookbook includes a range of tasty recipes that support digestive health and improve the quality of life for people with diverticulosis, with an emphasis on high-fiber, nutrient-dense foods.

The Power of Nutrition: Maintaining good nutrition is essential for treating diverticulosis. An effective food plan can have a big impact on how the condition progresses, how severe the symptoms are, how often they flare up, and how well a person feels overall. The secret to nutrition's potency is its capacity to both mitigate risk factors that could worsen symptoms of diverticulosis and supply the body with vital nutrients.

Impact of Diet on Diverticulosis: Diverticulosis is directly influenced by dietary practices in terms of both its onset and progression. Fruits, vegetables, whole grains, legumes, and other foods high in dietary fiber encourage regular bowel movements and ward against constipation, which lowers the risk of diverticular problems including infection and inflammation. On the other hand, a diet heavy in processed foods and poor in fiber may make diverticulitis episodes more likely because of the longer transit time through the colon and decreased volume of the stool.

Function of Nutrients in Relieving Symptoms: A number of nutrients are essential for reducing diverticulosis-related symptoms. Both soluble and insoluble fiber give feces more volume, which helps them travel through the colon more easily and lowers pressure inside the digestive system. Furthermore, keeping soft, passable stools is crucial for avoiding diverticular problems, which can be avoided with proper hydration. Some nutrients, such as vitamin E and omega-3 fatty acids, have anti-inflammatory qualities that may help reduce colon inflammation.

Pros of Antioxidant-Rich, Low-Carb, and Anti-Inflammatory Meals: For those who suffer from diverticulosis, a diet high in these nutrients has several advantages. Meals low in carbohydrates can help control blood sugar levels and avoid spikes that could make symptoms worse. Antioxidants, which are rich in fruits, vegetables, and some herbs and spices, help the body fight inflammation and oxidative stress, which may lower the chance of diverticular problems. In a similar vein, anti-inflammatory foods including leafy greens, nuts, seeds, and fatty fish can help reduce colon inflammation and alleviate symptoms while also improving gut health.

The significance of a balanced diet lies in its ability to guarantee that people with diverticulosis acquire enough nutrients while reducing the possibility of triggering symptoms. All nutrient-dense foods from the food groups should be included in a balanced diet, but a focus should be placed on foods high in fiber, such as fruits, vegetables, whole grains, and legumes. Lean proteins, good fats, and complex carbohydrates give the body the resources it needs to perform at its best, supporting general health and well-being.

How to Make Dietary Adjustments Sustainable: Creating long-lasting dietary adjustments requires implementing tactics that are doable and practical. Gradual changes are frequently easier to implement into daily life and more sustainable than large-scale overhauls. A person can monitor their progress and maintain motivation by setting clear, quantifiable goals, such as increasing fiber intake by consuming one more serving of fruits or vegetables each day. Finding tasty and entertaining dishes that follow dietary guidelines can also help to gradually make the switch to a diverticulosis-friendly diet more bearable and lasting. Long-term effectiveness in controlling diverticulosis through dietary interventions requires routine monitoring and modifications depending on individual preferences and responses.

CHAPTER TWO
Introducing the Diverticulosis Management

Diverticula, which are tiny pouches seen in the colon's walls, is a defining feature of diverticulosis. Diverticulitis, an inflammation or infection of these pouches, can result from diverticulosis, even though the condition may not exhibit any symptoms at all. Dietary changes that promote gut health and avoid flare-ups are the mainstay of diverticulosis management. We'll go over the crucial actions you need to take to get started on the path to successful diet-based diverticulosis management in this chapter.

Evaluating Your Current Diet: It's critical to comprehend how nutrition plays a part in managing diverticulosis. Evaluating your present eating patterns serves as a basis for implementing the required adjustments. It entails looking at the kinds of foods you often eat, your eating habits, and the portions you take. Do you eat adequate fiber? Do you often eat dairy products, red meat, or processed foods? Finding these features aids in determining where work has to be done.

Knowing What Foods to Avoid: Some foods can cause diverticulitis flare-ups or worsen the symptoms of diverticulosis. Nuts, seeds, popcorn, and high-fat foods are common trigger foods. By becoming stuck in the diverticula and creating irritation or inflammation, these objects have the potential to worsen symptoms associated with diverticular disease. One of the most important things in effectively controlling diverticulosis is identifying and avoiding trigger foods.

Knowing What You Eat Is Not Enough to Understand Your Dietary Patterns: There is more to understanding your eating patterns than that. It entails analyzing your eating surroundings, meal schedule, and emotional triggers for overindulging in food or choosing unhealthy options. Understanding your eating patterns will help you create plans for making adjustments that will improve your digestive system and general health.

Maintaining a Food Journal: Maintaining a food journal is a useful tool for monitoring your dietary consumption and any related symptoms. It is possible to find patterns and correlations between particular foods and flare-ups of symptoms by keeping a journal of everything you eat and drink, as well as any symptoms you feel. A food journal offers useful data that can direct dietary adjustments catered to your specific requirements.

Identifying Problematic Symptoms: Diverticulosis symptoms can differ greatly from person to person, and some people may not have any symptoms at all. However, bloating, rectal bleeding, altered bowel habits, and stomach pain are typical signs. For appropriate assessment and treatment, it's critical to pay attention to any odd or persistent symptoms and seek the advice of a healthcare provider.

Speaking with a Healthcare Professional: Although food changes are important for managing diverticulosis, you should see a healthcare provider, such as a qualified dietitian or gastroenterologist. Based on your nutritional preferences, unique needs, and medical history, they can offer tailored advice. Speaking with a healthcare provider will guarantee that you get all the attention and assistance you need to properly manage your illness.

In conclusion, implementing a diverticulosis management diet entails evaluating your present diet, determining trigger foods, comprehending your eating patterns, maintaining a food journal, identifying troubling symptoms, and speaking with a medical expert. You may minimize the risk of diverticular problems and improve your digestive health by being proactive and adopting educated food decisions.

Creating a Nutritious Plate: Creating a nutritious plate guarantees that you are receiving the proper ratio of nutrients to promote digestive health and general well-being, which is crucial for controlling diverticulosis. Typically, a well-rounded plate includes a range of food groups, such as whole grains, fruits, vegetables, lean proteins, and healthy fats. You can give your body the nutrients it needs to operate at its best by including these ingredients in your meals.

Including Foods High in Fibre: Fibre helps control bowel movements and prevents constipation, which can aggravate symptoms of diverticulosis. As such, it is an essential part of a diet for managing the illness. Fruits, vegetables, whole grains, legumes, and nuts are among the foods high in dietary fiber. By adding volume to the stool, these meals facilitate passage and lessen the chance of diverticula becoming infected or inflamed. To make sure you're getting a sufficient intake, try to include a range of fiber-rich foods in your meals and snacks throughout the day.

Selecting Lean Protein Sources: Lean protein sources offer the essential amino acids required for tissue maintenance and repair without contributing excess saturated fat, which can worsen inflammation. This makes them crucial for managing diverticulosis. Choose lean protein sources including fish, tofu, skinless chicken, lentils, and lean beef or pork chops. These choices can improve overall well-being and muscular health because they include less saturated fat.

Choosing Healthy Fats: Because they include vital fatty acids that promote cell growth and lower inflammation, healthy fats are a crucial component of a diet for managing diverticulosis. Choose high-fat foods like avocados, nuts, seeds, olive oil, and fatty fish like trout and salmon as your supplies of good fats. These fats can lessen the chance of flare-ups of diverticulitis and aid with bowel function.

Consuming a Wide Variety of Fruits and Vegetables: Fruits and vegetables are a great source of fiber, vitamins, minerals, and antioxidants, all of which are important for the management of diverticulosis. When planning meals and snacks, try to incorporate a selection of vibrant fruits and vegetables to make sure you're getting a variety of nutrients. By including fruits and vegetables in your diet, you can improve general digestive health, encourage regular bowel movements, and reduce inflammation.

Balancing Macronutrients: Diverticulosis management and general health depend on the proper balance of macronutrients, which include proteins, lipids, and carbs. Every meal should have a combination of carbohydrates, proteins, and fats to give your body long-lasting energy and support different body functions. Select complex carbs to help stabilize blood sugar levels and encourage fullness, such as whole grains, lean proteins, and healthy fats.

CHAPTER THREE

A Simple Guide to Meal Planning

Making a Weekly Meal Plan: For diverticulosis to be properly managed by diet, a weekly meal plan must be created. It permits deliberate meal selections that support digestive health and provide a balanced diet. First, think about the diverticulosis dietary guidelines, which usually call for high-fiber meals like fruits, vegetables, whole grains, and legumes. While considering dietary limitations and personal taste preferences, plan meals that feature these foods.

To keep things interesting and provide a good mix of nutrients, try to incorporate variation into your weekly meal plan. Add a variety of proteins, including fish, poultry, lentils, lean meats, and tofu. Add a variety of vibrant fruits and vegetables to your diet to offer a range of antioxidants, vitamins, and minerals.

To increase fiber consumption and promote digestive health, make a plan to eat whole grains such as quinoa, brown rice, and whole wheat pasta.

Meal Preparation in Advance: Think about making meals ahead of time to save time and follow your weekly meal plan. This could entail cooking in bulk on the weekends or on specific weekdays. Prepare significant quantities of basic items that may be used for several meals over the week, such as grains, proteins, and vegetables.

To safely keep prepared ingredients and meals in the refrigerator or freezer, make an investment in high-quality food storage containers. During hectic workdays, prepare meals ahead of time by chopping veggies, portioning snacks, and assembling components. Preparing meals ahead of time not only saves time but also lessens the temptation to choose convenience foods that aren't as healthful.

Selecting Convenient dishes: It's critical to select dishes that are both nutrient-dense and easy to make when controlling diverticulosis. Seek for recipes that call for few ingredients and easy preparation methods. Recipes for sheet pan dinners, slow cookers, and one-pot meals can be very practical because they need less cleanup and hands-on cooking time.

Make use of kitchen tools such as air fryers, blenders, and pressure cookers to speed up meal prep without compromising on nutrition. Select recipes that are flexible enough to accommodate your dietary requirements and tastes, whether that means making ingredient substitutions or changing the serving sizes.

Using Leftovers: If you're on a diverticulosis management diet, leftovers might be a great resource. Utilize leftover food to create fresh dinners or snacks rather than throwing it away. Leftover roasted vegetables, for instance, are great in grain bowls, soups, and salads. Grains that have been cooked, such as brown rice or quinoa, can be used to stuff peppers or make stir-fries.

Use leftovers in inventive ways by preparing them as wraps, sandwiches, or omelets. Remaining proteins, such as fish or grilled chicken, can be used for pasta meals or salads. Utilizing leftovers helps you maintain a diversified diet, save time and money, and minimize food waste.

Including Variation in Your Diet: A well-balanced and pleasurable diet is essential for managing diverticulosis. Try to eat a variety of meals from every food category to make sure you're getting a good range of nutrients. To keep meals interesting and fulfilling, try experimenting with new cooking techniques, flavor profiles, and cultural cuisines.

As long as they fit within your dietary requirements and constraints, don't be scared to try new meals or substances. Use seasonal produce to benefit from its fresh flavors and nutritional value. A variety of plant- and animal-based foods, such as beans, lentils, tofu, and seafood, should be included in your protein intake.

Taken together, these tactics for meal planning, cooking, choosing recipes, using leftovers, and varying your diet will help you control diverticulosis while still eating tasty and nourishing meals.

Purchasing Wisely:

The secret to controlling diverticulosis with diet is to shop wisely. Making informed decisions when shopping for groceries can have a big impact on your ability to follow a diet for managing diverticulosis and supporting digestive health in general. Here are some key ideas to think about:

Examining Nutrition Labels:
Anyone dealing with diverticulosis has to know how to read food labels. Seek foods that are low in saturated fats and added sugars and high in fiber. Serve portions with caution, and keep an eye out for any ingredients—like seeds or nuts—that could aggravate the illness or cause symptoms. By choosing foods that promote your digestive health, reading food labels gives you the power to make educated decisions about what you put into your body.

Selecting Whole Foods Instead of Processed Foods:

Whole foods are the best options for a diverticulosis treatment diet since they are little processed and still contain their natural nutrients. Your grocery list should be built around lean meats, whole grains, fresh produce, and healthy fats. Conversely, a lot of added sugars, preservatives, and other substances found in processed foods can aggravate the digestive tract and cause flare-ups. You may minimize the chance of stomach discomfort while providing your body with the necessary nutrients by making whole foods a priority.

Perimeter Shopping at the Grocery Store:
Sticking to the grocery store's perimeter is one easy way to shop wisely. The freshest, least processed produce, meats, dairy products, and whole grains can all be found

here. You can resist the urge to buy processed snacks and convenience foods that might not support your diverticulosis treatment objectives by concentrating your shopping efforts on these areas. Furthermore, shopping the perimeter motivates you to increase the amount of nutrient-dense items in your diet, which can improve your digestive system's general health.

Purchasing Necessary Pantry Items

Keeping diverticulosis-friendly staples in your cupboard guarantees that you'll always have wholesome options available. High-fiber cereals, whole-grain pasta and rice, canned beans, low-sodium broth, canned tomatoes, and unsweetened applesauce are a few cupboard mainstays to take into account. These adaptable components can serve as the foundation for a variety of dishes and snacks, which will make it simpler to follow your diet even on hectic days. You may make shopping easier and better prepare yourself for condition management by preemptively stocking up on pantry necessities.

Putting Up a Shopping List

Finally, spend some time creating a thorough grocery list before you go shopping. Arrange your weekly menu and note any ingredients you will need to buy. You may prevent impulsive buys and make sure you get home with everything you need to support your diverticulosis management diet by going shopping with a list. To further streamline your shopping experience, think about grouping items on your list according to food categories. You can shop with confidence in the supermarket aisles when you have a well-thought-out list in hand, knowing that the decisions you make will put your digestive health first.

In conclusion, wise purchasing is a crucial part of managing diverticulosis effectively. You can make sure that your grocery shopping visits support your dietary objectives and encourage optimal digestive health by reading food labels, selecting whole foods, stocking up on pantry basics, browsing the perimeter of the store, and creating a complete grocery list.

Cookbook for Managing Diverticulosis Diet

CHAPTER FOUR
Overcoming Obstacles

Handling desires: When using nutrition to treat diverticulosis, cravings can pose a serious problem. People often have cravings for high-fiber foods, which might make their condition worse. But giving in to these desires can make symptoms worse and cause discomfort. Finding healthy substitutes for cravings that satiate the same need is one way to manage them. For instance, choose fruits or vegetables that are easy on the stomach but nonetheless have a delightful crunch rather than processed food. Adding savory herbs and spices to food is another way to sate appetites without sacrificing nutrition. It's crucial to keep in mind that cravings are fleeting and frequently go away when the body becomes accustomed to a new eating pattern.

 Diverticulosis sufferers may have particular difficulties in social settings, particularly when dining out or going to events where dietary needs may not be well known. It's critical to prepare ahead of time and let friends, family, or restaurant personnel know about your dietary requirements in order to handle these circumstances successfully.

Think about recommending eateries that have menu items that are appropriate for your condition or offering to bring a dish to share that complies with your dietary needs. Additionally, you may make sure that your dietary concerns are acknowledged without needless conflict by being assertive about what you require while still being kind. Keep in mind that putting your health first is crucial, especially in social situations, and that having understanding friends and family who can support you and take care of your needs can really help.

Handling setbacks: Diverticulosis is a chronic ailment, and addressing it comes with setbacks. Setbacks can be demoralizing and disappointing, regardless of the cause—a momentary break in dietary adherence or a flare-up of symptoms. On the other hand, it's critical to face obstacles with self-compassion and patience. Instead of focusing on what went wrong, consider what you can take away from the experience and how to avoid making the same mistakes again. This could entail going over your diet plan again, figuring out what causes your symptoms, or getting advice from a medical expert. Recall that obstacles are a chance for development and adaptation rather than a sign of failure.

Asking for help from loved ones: Having loved ones' support can be very helpful in controlling diverticulosis. Having a solid support network can substantially impact your journey, whether it be in the form of emotional support, useful aid with meal preparation, or just someone to listen to. Never be afraid to ask friends, family, or support groups for assistance and motivation when you need it. Openly discuss your illness and how your loved ones can best support you with them. Sometimes, it can be incredibly relieving to know that you're not the only one going through difficult circumstances, and it can also serve as a great inspiration to stick to your management plan.

Maintaining motivation: It can be difficult to maintain motivation to follow a diverticulosis management diet, particularly when faced with temptations or disappointments. Consider the advantages of dietary modifications for your overall health and well-being as a means of maintaining your motivation. Remind yourself of the advantages of eating a low-residue, high-fiber diet, including better digestive health and a decreased chance of flare-ups.

Maintaining accountability and motivation can also be achieved by setting reasonable goals and monitoring your advancement. Appreciate the little things that go right along the way, like trying a new cuisine that works for your diverticulosis or getting through a social gathering without feeling uncomfortable. Lastly, develop a resilient and self-compassionate mindset, understanding that diverticulosis management is a journey that calls for perseverance and commitment but ultimately results in improved health and quality of life.

Smoothies high in fiber: Smoothies are a great way to start the day with a good dose of fiber and nutrition. This section's recipes focus on using foods like fruits, vegetables, and seeds that are high in soluble and insoluble fiber. For instance, spinach, kale, banana, avocado, and flaxseeds mixed with almond milk or Greek yogurt for creaminess may make up a traditional green smoothie. These components include important vitamins, minerals, and antioxidants to support gut health in addition to a significant amount of fiber.

Muesli with fruits and nuts: Muesli is a popular breakfast food that is great for those with diverticulosis because of its high fiber content.

 The recipes in this section are centered around

adding fresh fruits and nuts to muesli to improve its nutritional value. To add texture and heart-healthy lipids, a recipe can call for cooking steel-cut oats with diced apples, cinnamon, and a sprinkling of almonds or walnuts. These muesli recipes increase fiber consumption, supply vital nutrients, and encourage satiety throughout the morning by combining a range of fruits and nuts.

Vegetable omelets: Eggs are a flexible, high-protein food that can be included in a breakfast that is suitable for diverticulosis. Breakfast dishes like vegetable omelets are a filling and tasty way to add more fiber to your diet. Often, a range of vibrant veggies, including tomatoes, onions, bell peppers, and spinach, are sautéed till soft and then combined with fluffy eggs in these dishes. These omelets improve digestive health and symptom management in addition to adding texture and flavor by combining veggies high in fiber.

Greek yogurt parfaits: Known for its high protein content and probiotic qualities, Greek yogurt is a wholesome breakfast choice. For those with diverticulosis, Greek yogurt parfaits provide a quick and filling dinner option. Greek yogurt is usually layered with crunchy like granola or chopped almonds, and fresh fruits like diced mango, sliced bananas, or berries. Probiotics from Greek yogurt help maintain gut health, and fiber-rich fruits and nuts give vital nutrients that assist regular digestion and general wellness.

Whole grain pancakes: By choosing recipes that use whole grain flour and include extra fiber-rich toppings components, pancakes can still be enjoyed as part of a diet that is favorable to diverticulosis. Pancakes made with whole grains are a healthy take on a traditional breakfast staple, including vital nutrients and a substantial amount of dietary fiber. Whole wheat flour or oat flour may be the foundation of these recipes, with additional ingredients such as ground flaxseeds to increase fiber content or mashed bananas or grated zucchini. For those who are managing diverticulosis, these pancakes provide a tasty and nutritious breakfast alternative whether topped with fresh fruit or drizzled with honey.

All things considered, the breakfast recipes found in Chapter 2 of the "Diverticulosis Management Diet Cookbook" are meant to offer wholesome choices that promote intestinal health and help control symptoms. These recipes provide tasty ways to start the day on the right foot while boosting general well-being for people with diverticulosis since they emphasize nutritious foods and ingredients that are high in fiber.

Quinoa: Packed with fiber and adaptable, quinoa is a great whole-grain option for people with diverticulitis. Those who suffer from diverticulosis benefit from its high fiber content, which facilitates digestion and helps avoid constipation.

veggies: Adding a range of vibrant veggies to the salad boosts its nutritional value and flavor. Leafy greens, bell peppers, cucumbers, tomatoes, and carrots are just a few examples of vegetables that are full of vital vitamins, minerals, and antioxidants that help with digestion and general health.

Dressing: You can improve the flavor of the salad without adding too many calories or fat by using a light vinaigrette dressing made with olive oil, lemon juice, or balsamic vinegar.

CHAPTER FIVE

Avocado and Turkey Wraps

Turkey: People with diverticulosis typically handle lean proteins like turkey well and they're a wonderful source of nutrients. Turkey offers the high-quality protein that's needed to maintain muscle mass and heal damaged tissue without adding too much-saturated fat.

Avocado: Avocado gives the wrap a nice dose of fiber and adds creaminess and healthy fats. Avocados include heart-healthy monounsaturated fats that can lower cholesterol.

Whole Grain Wraps: Choosing whole grain tortillas or wraps increases the amount of fiber in the meal, which helps to maintain digestive

Leafy Greens: Including leafy greens in the wrap, such as kale or spinach, increases its vitamin and fiber content and gives it a delightful crunch and freshness.

Soup with Lentils:

Lentils: Packed with fiber, protein, and a variety of vitamins and minerals, lentils are a nutritional powerhouse. Their high fiber content helps avoid constipation, which is a typical issue for people with diverticulosis and encourages regular bowel movements.

Broth Base: To add flavor without going overboard with sodium, use a vegetable or low-sodium chicken broth as the soup's base. This will help you keep your blood pressure levels in check.

Vegetables: Adding veggies to the soup, such as carrots, celery, onions, and tomatoes, boosts its fiber and nutritional value while also improving its flavor.

Herbs and Spices: The soup becomes flavorful and nutrient-dense by adding herbs and spices like paprika, cumin, thyme, and garlic. This is done without using too much salt.

Grilled Caesar Salad with Chicken:

Grilled Chicken: A diet plan for managing diverticulosis must include lean protein sources like grilled chicken breast. Chicken that has been grilled gains flavor without gaining additional fat, making it a filling and healthful choice.

Romaine Lettuce: Diverticulosis sufferers typically tolerate romaine lettuce well because it is a low-fiber veggie. It's the perfect base for a Caesar salad because of its mild flavor and crisp texture.

Homemade Caesar Dressing: Creating your own Caesar dressing gives you more control over the components, especially the fat and salt content. Greek yogurt or a low-fat mayonnaise can be used as a basis to help save fat and calories without sacrificing texture.

Whole Grain Croutons: By omitting refined grains, which could worsen diverticulosis symptoms, whole grain croutons give the salad more fiber and crunch.

Stir-fried vegetables with tofu:

Tofu: Rich in protein and low in saturated fat, tofu is a versatile plant-based protein that's a fantastic choice for people who have diverticulosis. It gives the essential amino acids required for maintaining and repairing muscle without unduly taxing the digestive tract.

Assorted Vegetables: Stir-frying a range of vibrant veggies, such as carrots, bell peppers, broccoli, snap peas, and mushrooms, boosts the dish's fiber and nutritional value in addition to adding taste and texture.

Low-Sodium Sauce: Using a homemade stir-fry sauce or low-sodium soy sauce helps you better regulate how much sodium you eat, which is crucial for blood pressure management and lowering your risk of diverticulosis complications.

Whole Grain Brown Rice or Quinoa: This dish provides more fiber and complex carbs to the stir-fry, which helps to maintain digestive health and gives you energy for a longer period of time.

A diverticulosis management diet cookbook can help people eat tasty and nourishing meals that promote their overall health and digestive health by concentrating on these lunch ideas.

Salmon baked in a pan with roasted veggies:

Salmon: Due to its anti-inflammatory qualities, omega-3 fatty acids, which are abundant in salmon, may help lessen the inflammation brought on by diverticulosis. Moreover, it contains a lot of protein, which is necessary for both general health and tissue repair.

Roasted veggies: Roasting veggies intensifies their flavor and brings out their inherent sweetness. Because they are rich in fiber, vitamins, and minerals, vegetables like bell peppers, carrots, and zucchini are good for your digestive system and general health. For those who have diverticulosis, constipation is a typical worry that can be avoided with the aid of fiber.

Marinara Sauce over Spaghetti Squash: Spaghetti squash: If you're on a diverticulosis management diet, spaghetti squash is a healthy substitute for regular pasta. It is easy on the stomach because it is rich in fiber and low in calories and carbs. Spaghetti squash contains soluble fiber, which helps maintain intestinal regularity and may lessen diverticulosis symptoms.

Marinara Sauce: Spaghetti squash tastes great with homemade marinara sauce. Choosing a sauce produced with fresh tomatoes, onions, garlic, and herbs guarantees that it is devoid of additives and preservatives that could exacerbate gastrointestinal distress. Antioxidants found in abundance in tomatoes, such as lycopene, may have anti-inflammatory properties and improve digestive health.

Beef: Lean beef cuts are a rich source of important minerals like zinc and iron as well as protein. Mealtime protein intake increases satiety and stabilizes blood sugar, both of which are advantageous for those with diverticulosis. To reduce your intake of saturated fat, which is detrimental to your heart health, choose lean beef cuts.

Broccoli: Packed full of vitamins, minerals, and fiber, broccoli is a cruciferous vegetable. Because it has a significant amount of fiber, it helps to maintain regular bowel motions and stave against constipation. Sulforaphane, one of the substances found in broccoli, is thought to have anti-inflammatory qualities and improve gut health in general.

Bell peppers that are stuffed:

Bell peppers: Packed with antioxidants that enhance immune system function and improve skin health, bell peppers are low in calories and high in vitamins A and C. They also include a good amount of fiber, which promotes healthy digestion and may help avoid issues like diverticulitis caused by diverticulosis. A flexible and wholesome dinner choice that can be tailored to each person's taste preferences is stuffed bell peppers.

Filling Options: When making stuffed bell peppers, take into account packing them full of veggies, nutritious grains, and lean protein. A filling consisting of quinoa, black beans, maize, and spices, for instance, offers a gratifying blend of flavor, protein, and fiber. Eating a choice of vibrant veggies guarantees a varied spectrum of nutrients and phytochemicals that promote general health.

Pizza with Cauliflower Crust:

Cauliflower Crust: Suitable for people with celiac disease or gluten intolerance, cauliflower crust pizza provides a gluten-free substitute for typical wheat-based pizza dough. While cauliflower is low in calories and carbs, it is high in fiber and essential minerals like vitamins K and C. Adding an extra serving of vegetables to the meal by using cauliflower as the base for the pizza dough is good for the health of the digestive system.

Toppings: Use nutrient-dense foods like tomato sauce, lean protein (like turkey sausage or grilled chicken), and a range of veggies (including spinach, mushrooms, and bell peppers) to top pizza made with cauliflower crust. Reducing the amount of processed and high-fat toppings, such as sausage and pepperoni, can help lower the chance of making diverticulosis symptoms worse.

Dip with Carrot Sticks:

A tasty and healthful spread, hummus is mostly made of chickpeas, lemon juice, garlic, and tahini (sesame seed paste). It is high in fiber, several vitamins and minerals, and plant-based protein. Because of its high fiber content, which supports regular bowel movements and digestive health, hummus can be helpful for people managing diverticulosis when added to their diet.

Hummus and vegetable sticks, like bell peppers, carrots, celery, and cucumbers, go well together and provide additional fiber, vitamins, and minerals to the snack. These veggies are satisfying and hydrating because they are high in water content and low in calories. It's also a tasty snack option because the crunchiness of the vegetables offers a pleasing tactile contrast to the creamy hummus.

For people with diverticulosis, whole-grain crackers are the better option because they include more fiber than refined-grain crackers. In order to manage diverticulosis, fiber aids avoid constipation and support overall digestive health. Whole grain crackers also include complex carbs, which digest more slowly and result in longer-lasting energy and improved blood sugar regulation.

Made from almonds, which are high in fiber, protein, vitamins, and minerals, almond butter is a wholesome spread. It's a great source of monounsaturated fats, which have been linked to a number of health advantages, such as less inflammation and a better heart. The high fiber content of almond butter helps to maintain regular bowel movements and digestive health, making it a good addition to the diet for people who suffer from diverticulosis.

Almond butter and whole grain crackers combine to provide a snack that is more satisfying and full by adding more fiber, protein, and complex carbs. The mild nutty flavor and crunchy texture of whole-grain crackers balance out the richness of the almond butter. Furthermore, because whole grain crackers include more fiber and nutrients—both of which are critical for digestive health and general well-being—than refined grain crackers, they are a healthier option.

Selecting almond butter requires making sure that it doesn't contain hydrogenated oils or added sugars, as these ingredients can be harmful to health, particularly for those who have diverticulosis. Choose almond butter that is natural or organic, manufactured solely of almonds, and devoid of any additional substances. Additionally, because nut butter is high in calories, portion control is essential while eating it. Adhere to the suggested portion size in order to prevent overindulgence and preserve a balanced intake of nutrients.

High in protein, calcium, and probiotics, Greek yogurt is a dairy product that is packed with nutrients. Probiotics are good bacteria that support gut health by preserving a balanced population of microbes in the digestive system. Probiotic-rich foods, such as Greek yogurt, can help maintain digestive health and relieve symptoms like gas, bloating, and constipation in people with diverticulosis.

Berries are a great source of vitamins, minerals, antioxidants, and fiber. Examples of these include raspberries, blackberries, blueberries, and strawberries. They are satisfying and hydrating because they have a high water content and few calories. Berries are also a great source of dietary fiber, which helps avoid constipation—a typical problem for people with diverticulosis—and encourages regular bowel movements.

Berries and Greek yogurt combine to make a tasty and nourishing snack that is ideal for those with diverticulosis. Fresh berries' acidic and sweet flavors blend beautifully with Greek yogurt's creamy texture to create a delightful and revitalizing treat. Greek yogurt and berries also contain protein, probiotics, fiber, and antioxidants, which together offer a host of other health advantages like better immune system performance, less inflammation, and improved digestion.

Select Greek yogurts that are pure and unsweetened, free of artificial ingredients or added sugars. High levels of added sugars are frequently found in flavored yogurts, which can be harmful to health, particularly in those who have diverticulosis. Rather than using additional sugars, use fresh or frozen berries to naturally sweeten your Greek yogurt. Berries contribute sweetness, flavor, and minerals.

Slices of apple with peanut butter:
Apples are nutrient-dense fruit that is rich in antioxidants, fiber, vitamins, and minerals. In addition, they are low in calories and high in soluble fiber, which lowers blood sugar and increases sensations of fullness and satiety. Because apples are high in fiber, including them in the diet can help maintain digestive health and reduce constipation for those with diverticulosis.

Roasted peanuts are used to make peanut butter, a popular spread that is high in protein, vitamins, and minerals, as well as good fats. It's a great source of monounsaturated fats, which have been linked to a number of health advantages, such as less inflammation and a better heart. Because of its high fiber content and satiating qualities, peanut butter can be a beneficial addition to the diet for those who suffer from diverticulosis.

Apple slices and peanut butter combine to make a tasty and wholesome snack that is ideal for those with diverticulosis. This delightful and full meal is made possible by the natural sweetness and crunchiness of apples combined with the creamy and nutty flavor of peanut butter. In addition, the fiber, protein, and good fats in apples and peanut butter help maintain stable blood sugar levels and offer long-lasting energy.

Choose natural or organic peanut butter that is produced solely of peanuts and doesn't contain any added sugars, hydrogenated oils, or artificial components. Steer clear of peanut butter that has partially hydrogenated oils or additional salt since these additives might be harmful to your health, especially if you have diverticulosis. Adhere to the suggested portion size in order to prevent overindulgence and preserve a balanced intake of nutrients.

Nuts and dried fruits in a trail mix:

A handy and transportable snack, trail mix is composed of a blend of nuts, seeds, dried fruits, and occasionally chocolate or granola. Being rich in protein, fiber, healthy fats, vitamins, minerals, and antioxidants, it's a nutrient-dense choice for people with diverticulosis. To fit your nutritional requirements and tastes, you must, however, carefully select the ingredients for your trail mix.

Nuts are a great source of protein, fiber, vitamins, minerals, and healthy fats. Some examples of nuts are cashews, walnuts, almonds, and pistachios. They also include a lot of antioxidants, which lower inflammation in the body and shield cells from harm from free radicals. Because nuts have high fiber content, they can help maintain digestive health and reduce constipation for people with diverticulosis.

Dried fruits are concentrated sources of vitamins, minerals, fiber, and antioxidants. Examples of these fruits are raisins, apricots, cranberries, and cherries. They're a great addition to trail mix because they're naturally sweet and offer immediate energy. But because dried fruits have more sugar and calories than fresh fruits, it's important to eat them in moderation. To prevent overindulgence and preserve a balanced intake of nutrients, stick to modest serving sizes.

When creating trail mix for people with diverticulosis, it's important to include a range of dried fruits and nuts that don't contain added sugars or artificial additives. For additional fiber, protein, and omega-3 fatty acids, you can also add seeds, such as chia, pumpkin, and sunflower seeds. Steer clear of adding chocolate or sugar-filled granola, as these might be harmful to your health, especially if you have diverticulosis. For a healthier snack choice, go with dark chocolate or unsweetened granola.

Fruit salad, especially with a zesty honey-lime dressing, is a delicious and revitalizing way to cap off a meal. Because of the variety of fruits used, this dish is not only delicious but also nutrient-dense, offering a range of vitamins, minerals, and antioxidants.

Fibre Content: Fruit salad can be a great complement to a diverticulosis management diet, especially when made with high-fiber fruits like berries, apples, and oranges. Because it prevents constipation and encourages regular bowel movements, fiber can help heal diverticulosis symptoms and support a healthy digestive system.

Low in Added Sugar: Natural honey can be used to make the honey-lime dressing, adding sweetness without using a lot of added sugar. For those who have diverticulosis, controlling sugar intake is essential because excessive sugar consumption can aggravate symptoms and increase intestinal inflammation.

Hydration: Fruits naturally contain water, which can help with hydration, a crucial component of managing diverticulosis. Maintaining adequate hydration lowers the risk of problems like diverticulitis by softening and making it easier to pass stool.

Antioxidants: Vitamin C and flavonoids, two types of antioxidants abundant in fruits, aid in the body's fight against oxidative stress and inflammation. Consuming a diet high in antioxidant-rich foods can improve digestive health in general and lower the chance of diverticulosis flare-ups.

Pudding with Chia Seeds:

Chia seed pudding is a healthy and adaptable dessert choice that may be made to fit personal tastes. Chia seeds are soaked in liquid (milk or a dairy-free substitute) until they take on the consistency of gel. This custard is a nice treat for people on a diverticulosis management diet since it may be sweetened and flavored in a variety of ways.

Omega-3 Fatty Acids: Rich in anti-inflammatory qualities, plant-based omega-3 fatty acids are found in chia seeds. Consuming foods high in omega-3 fatty acids can help minimize gastrointestinal tract inflammation and potentially minimize the chance of flare-ups of diverticulitis.

Rich in Fibre: Chia seeds are a great source of fiber, which is good for the health of your digestive system. Fiber avoids constipation, encourages regular bowel movements, and gives stool more volume—all of which are crucial factors to take into account when managing diverticulosis.

Texture Modification: Chia seed pudding may be a good choice for people with diverticulosis who may need to stay away from certain textures that can irritate their digestive systems. Those with sensitive digestive systems may find the soft, gel-like texture to be well-tolerated as it is mild on the intestines.

Natural Sweeteners: You can use mashed fruit or maple syrup in place of refined sugars when sweetening chia seed pudding. This helps to keep blood sugar levels steady and lowers the chance of aggravating diverticulosis symptoms.

Dipped Strawberries in Dark Chocolate:

Strawberries dipped in dark chocolate are a rich and relatively nutritious dessert option that blends the natural sweetness of strawberries with the antioxidant-rich qualities of dark chocolate.

Principles of the Diverticulosis Management Diet:

Antioxidant Benefits: Flavonoids, which are abundant in dark chocolate, are strong

Method of Management

High-Fiber Diet: A high-fiber diet helps prevent constipation and soften feces, which lessens the pressure on the colon walls and lowers the risk of inflammation and diverticula formation. It is imperative to include fruits, vegetables, whole grains, and legumes.

Hydration: It's critical to maintain healthy digestion and stave off constipation by consuming enough water. Try to drink eight glasses of water or more if you live in a hot area or are physically active.

Frequent Physical Activity: Exercise supports regular bowel motions and digestive health in general. Exercises like swimming, yoga, running, and walking can help with bowel movement and lower the risk of problems from diverticulosis.

CHAPTER SEVEN

How much fiber a day should I be getting

The amount of fiber that is advised daily varies based on age, gender, and general health. However, it's usually advised to strive for 25 to 35 grams of fiber per day for people who have diverticulosis. It's crucial to increase fiber consumption gradually to prevent uncomfortable digestive symptoms like gas or bloating.

Foods High in Fibre:

Fruits: oranges, pears, apples, and berries

Vegetables: Brussels sprouts, broccoli, carrots, and spinach

Whole Grains: whole wheat bread, brown rice, quinoa, and oats

Legumes: Chickpeas, lentils, and beans

Are there any foods that I should totally stay away from?

Diverticulosis sufferers may find that some foods make their symptoms worse or cause flare-ups, but there is no one-size-fits-all solution. Among them are:

Processed Foods: Processed foods with a lot of fat and sugar can aggravate the digestive system and cause inflammation. Restrict your consumption of processed meats, sugary snacks, and fried foods.

Low-Fiber Foods: Consuming low-fiber foods can cause constipation, which can exacerbate the symptoms of diverticulosis by putting more strain on the gut walls. White rice, packaged snacks, and bread should be avoided or consumed in moderation.

Nuts and Seeds: Although they were originally thought to pose a risk to people with diverticulosis, a new study indicates that this may not be the case. It's advisable to stay away from them, though, if you find they aggravate your symptoms.

Can I still indulge in goodies now and then?

When it comes to indulging in rare pleasures, moderation is essential. Diverticulosis management requires a healthy, high-fiber diet first and foremost, but occasionally treating yourself to indulgences is usually OK. However, it's important to watch portion sizes and frequency because eating too many unhealthy meals might upset your digestive system and perhaps cause symptoms.

How should I respond in the event of a flare-up?

Changes in bowel habits, bloating, and stomach pain are all possible signs of a diverticulosis flare-up. It's critical to take action to reduce symptoms and stop problems. What you can do is as follows:

Dietary Modifications: To give your digestive system a break and allow it to repair, temporarily stick to a low-fiber or clear liquid diet. Reintroduce meals high in fiber gradually when symptoms become better.

Hydration: To help with digestion and avoid dehydration, consume lots of fluids like water, herbal tea, or clear broths.

Over-the-Counter Drugs: Acetaminophen and other over-the-counter painkillers can help reduce discomfort. Ibuprofen and other nonsteroidal anti-inflammatory medicines (NSAIDs) should be avoided, though, as they might worsen symptoms and raise the possibility of problems.

Medical Evaluation: Seek immediate medical assistance if symptoms worsen or persist. To treat symptoms and avoid complications, your healthcare professional can advise additional testing or write a prescription for medicine.

In conclusion, although nutrition alone cannot cure diverticulosis, controlling symptoms and avoiding complications can be achieved by following certain guidelines, such as eating a high-fiber diet, drinking plenty of water, exercising frequently, and indulging in rare delicacies in moderation. It's also critical to recognize trigger foods and take the right action to properly control flare-ups. Seek additional assessment and advice from a healthcare provider if symptoms worsen or continue.

An Example of a Menu:

First Week:

First Day:

Berry and spinach smoothie for breakfast

Snack: Granola and berries paired with a Greek yogurt parfait

Lunch is Primavera Whole Grain Pasta.

Snack: A salad of fresh fruit

Steamed asparagus and baked salmon with lemon and dill for dinner

Day 2:

Omelette of vegetables for breakfast

Snack: Almonds

Brown rice with stir-fried turkey and vegetables for lunch

Snack: Hummus-topped carrot sticks

Black beans and Quinoa Stuffed Bell Peppers for Dinner

For the remainder of the week, stick to this routine, making sure to eat a combination of foods high in fiber, lean proteins, healthy fats, and lots of water.

"Soothing Recipes and Balanced Guidance for Managing Diverticulosis: A Holistic 7-Day Meal Plan to Promote Digestive Comfort and Optimal Wellness" is the meal plan's subtitle.

THE END

www.ingramcontent.com/pod-product-compliance
Lightning Source LLC
Chambersburg PA
CBHW061301250726
48653CB00002B/726